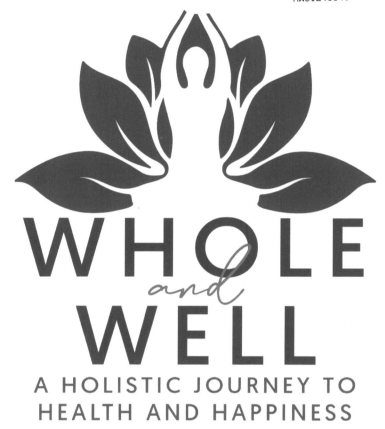

WHOLE *and* WELL

A HOLISTIC JOURNEY TO HEALTH AND HAPPINESS

Give Love and Attention to the whole body,
mind and soul to live a long, happy and healthy life!

KATHY E. N. PROCTOR
MS, BSN, RN, CCM

Disclaimer

The information provided in this book is intended for general informational and educational purposes only. It is not a substitute for professional medical advice, diagnosis, or treatment. Always seek the advice of your physician, healthcare provider, or other qualified health professionals with any questions you may have regarding a medical condition or before starting any new diet, exercise, or wellness program.

The author and publisher of this book are not responsible for any adverse effects or consequences resulting from the use of any suggestions, procedures, or dietary advice contained within this book. The content is based on the author's research, experiences, and opinions and is provided "as is" without any guarantees or warranties of any kind.

The reader assumes full responsibility for their health and well-being and agrees to use this information at their own risk. This book is not intended to diagnose, treat, cure, or prevent any disease, and any action taken based on the contents of this book should be undertaken after consultation with a healthcare professional.

By reading this book, you acknowledge that you have read, understood, and agree to this disclaimer.

ACKNOWLEDGMENT

I want to express my gratitude to God for the gift of teaching, nurturing, and helping others. I am thankful for the strength to continue my journey in life, health, and wellness. It was placed in my heart and my patients inspired me to write a book. This book aims to connect us and guide us back to the fundamentals of achieving wellness and optimal health, enabling us to live well regardless of the challenges we may encounter.

DEDICATIONS

This book is dedicated to the many lives that have transitioned to their next life but left a stamp in my heart and memory and were part of my healing and discovering my passion to advocate for holistic health practices.

Daddy, I was too young to understand what end-stage renal disease was and how it was going to take you away before having a chance to see you attend one more graduation, which is why I diverted from my plans of becoming a doctor and settled on being a nurse. I had no clue that God was still working to steer me into my destined career path through your illness. I thought this would be a quick way to graduate, but God saw the bigger picture. Anyhow, you were stubborn and refused dialysis, insisting that "I'm Muslim and ready to die and no one is going to cut you," but then, on one night of delirium and increased BUN, creatinine, potassium, and severely elevated BP, you were placed on emergency dialysis, which bought you more time on this earth and allowed us to make more memories. These memories are glued to my heart, mind, and soul so many years later. God heard and answered my prayers because on May 27, 2003, not only did I turn 22, but you were present at pinning and witnessed me take the oath to be the best darn nurse I can be. A week later, you were there to pick me up from work and asked, "Did you kill someone yet?" I loved your crazy sense of humor, although that question was nuts to ask, but that was your sense of humor. One year of these foolish questions, short to long drives, quick runs for lottery tickets, me telling you about the family after each visit to Antigua, and simply spending time with you until you received that transplant which you suddenly agreed to. However, Dad, you were my first lesson that we all will have and meet our final destination no matter how much we try to fight to prolong life. We have no control or know when our time is up, and your departure was the worst and my first experience with instant, unprepared death. I woke up with all of my windows, with the exception of the front and rear, shattered, but not one thing was stolen from my vehicle, which was bizarre. What was even more bizarre was the phone call from my mother saying you never came home last night! I searched and called everywhere, and the dialysis center stated you left without any issue, but then I received the worst call of my life, stating that you were struck by a car and are currently in ICU. I know deep in spirit that the shattered windows were your rage that I was all the way in Brooklyn with my old buddy while you were in the Bronx fighting to survive, or maybe holding on until I came. My buddy helped put some bags on my newly purchased car that you so happened to tell me not to purchase literally 2 months prior because you were big on saving for a house, and then I got the car. But you know your daughter was a free spirit and marched to her own beat just like you. I arrived and saw the involuntary movements and felt like your spirit was already traveling to a more peaceful place, and that is exactly what happened less than 48 hours after being hit by a car. My world shattered like your bones, my car windows, and broken car pieces that contributed to your sudden departure. I never imagined that I would say goodbye to my best friend, dad, protector, teacher, and first love at the age of 23, but I did, and it was the start of my depression but the beginning of a new chapter, rebirth, and a new life.

Depression led to a spiral of irresponsible behaviors that landed me with a positive pregnancy test and urinary urgency and the inability to keep my eyes open. I wish there was a bed and a commode everywhere I went because I couldn't stop running to urinate, and my eyes couldn't stay open for long. No nausea or any other symptoms, but I knew my plans to continue with my RN to BSN were going on a long pause so I could hustle and grind because I was going to be a single mom. That story has no place in this book, but I will discuss ways to identify and manage stressors, including people. I will also say that sometimes it is better to walk away and believe that the Lord will provide more than what the courts and human beings can.

My baby came via C-section, and that was a very interesting journey with a beautiful outcome and was surrounded by some amazing people who are no longer part of my current circle, but they all hold a special and permanent place in my heart, memories, and albums. That's one thing about me; I learned to cut dead branches but can never forget that they contributed to my growth, and they once bore leaves that bloomed in their season, but one day it stopped, and holding on was slowing my growth. So, we let go with no malice or hate, but with love. So, I dedicate this book to my sisters, and you know who you are. Just know that I will always love you all although we have separated to grow in another path.

Back to my daughter, and the bridge and catalyst, lovely sunshine, and a new heartbeat and teacher. You came to give me purpose again, and your birth led me to make many career changes that led me to discover my love for community health, especially caring for my Bronx people. I love the Bronx, and I love my people with my entire heart. Laynie, you are the bridge that connected my mother and me because we were like oil and water. Still, fortunately for you, I always felt like my experience may not be your experience, so I ensured you had a relationship with your grandma. However, my mother and I have been broken since I was ten years old. But baby girl, you were my mother's little star, a ray of sunshine, and her best friend. She loved you until her last breath. Anyhow, back to us, girl, we made it and traveled to many foreign and local places together; you are my travel buddy and passenger on a long road trip, my headache, and the reason I keep my running sneakers on standby. But honestly, you are my gift from God and the universe and a star that will leave your mark on this earth. I love and thank you, Laynie Janae.

To my patients, who became my family, some are now angels. Each of you helped me heal and recover from a devastating loss. I was too young to understand and help my father avoid the complications related to diabetes and hypertension. The health system failed to give him the support, education, and guidance to make informed decisions. Instead, they pumped him with any new or trial medications that are now contraindicated in people with renal disease. They did not offer natural and alternative options, but I had a chance to offer them to the community I served while working as a visiting nurse. One thing that my patients did not know is how impactful they were in my healing from grief, loss, and depression. Some have passed on, but they or their beautiful and loving families are my family forever.

To my daddy's family, all of you are the reason I travel to Antigua as often as possible to spend time, have some rum, and indulge in some fun relaxing times with my cousins. My aunties who have passed on, please know that I love you on earth and love you in the afterlife. The words of wisdom and infectious smiles are what I see when I close my eyes and think of each of you. To my Aunt Paulette, you remind me so much of my daddy and your big brother. I thank God that he picked you and the Proctors/Freemans to be my bloodline. I'm so proud of my roots and DNA.

Lastly, to my beloved mommy, you taught me how to fight and to never give up despite the odds. You made my life hell, and I was mad for a very long time, but not mad enough to keep me from fulfilling my assignment on earth and turning cold. You showed me a lot about holding on to the past and being resentful, and how it can turn into an illness that slowly strips you of the very things that you fought so hard to obtain. You also taught me to stop waiting for an apology from others and to apologize to myself for not forgiving a lot sooner. You taught me that parents do what they think is best in that present moment, even if their decisions have a negative impact on the child's life. You also taught me that you did your part, which was bringing me into this world, and because of that, I exist. Thank you for creating me and contributing to my craziness, but mainly to the amazing woman despite the early and middle story of my childhood. This will not be discussed in this book, but I may cover it in my next book. Let's see."

APPRECIATION

To the Amazing Readers,

Thank you for embarking on this transformative journey with me. This book is the culmination of my unwavering dedication to crafting a holistic recipe for a better life. It's a labor of love that has been fueled by my unwavering passion for health, wellness, and the pursuit of a balanced life.

As you turn the pages, I want you to feel empowered, uplifted, and inspired. My goal is to provide you with the tools and insights to nurture your mind, body, and soul. This book is not just a collection of words, but a guiding light that aims to help you realize your true potential, overcome obstacles, and embrace a life filled with vitality and joy.

I invite you to join me on this incredible voyage of self-discovery, as we uncover the timeless wisdom of natural and holistic healing. Together, let's cultivate a harmonious existence that radiates with positivity and well-being. This is not just a book, but a companion that will walk alongside you as you embark on the incredible journey to wellness and fulfillment.

With boundless gratitude and endless optimism,

Kathy Proctor,

CONTENTS

1.
INTRODUCTION

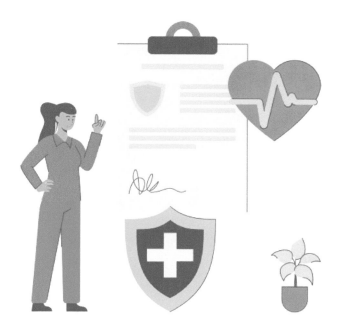

The Power of Taking Charge

I n today's fast-paced world, it's easy to feel like we have little control over our health. We often rely solely on doctors to solve our health issues without taking an active role in our own well-being. However, it's important to recognize that we have the power to make choices that significantly impact our health. Imagine a scenario where you and your doctor engage in meaningful conversations about your health. You share your experiences, concerns, and goals for a healthier life. Your doctor listens attentively, understands your unique story, and works with you to identify the root causes of any health issues. This kind of proactive communication can lead to more personalized and effective care, ultimately resulting in better outcomes and a stronger doctor-patient relationship.

The Role of Lifestyle in Health

Mainstream medicine often overlooks the impact of lifestyle on our well-being. However, the truth is that many illnesses stem from the choices we make in our daily lives. It's crucial for all of us to recognize the power we hold in making lifestyle changes that can help prevent the occurrence of various diseases.

A strong doctor-patient relationship is built on trust, open communication, and collaboration. When doctors take the time to truly understand their patients – not just their symptoms – and involve them in their care, patients feel heard, valued, and empowered. As a result, patients are more likely to adhere to their treatment plans and take an active role in their health.

Embracing Wholeness: Nurturing the Complete Self

Maintaining good health and wellness involves a comprehensive approach that encompasses various aspects of well-being. These aspects are intrinsically linked to our environment, lifestyle choices, and genetic predisposition, all of which play a critical role in shaping our overall health. A well-rounded diet rich in essential nutrients such as vitamin C, D, omega-3 fats, zinc, and probiotics is essential to support our body's functions and ward off the negative effects of unhealthy food choices. Engaging in a regular exercise regimen can significantly contribute to weight management, stress reduction, and the maintenance of optimal mental health. Prioritizing sufficient rest and sleep is crucial for overall well-being. Minimizing exposure to environmental toxins present in our food, cleaning supplies, and food containers is imperative. Finding fulfillment in purposeful work and setting and pursuing meaningful goals can greatly enhance our overall well-being. Cultivating a spirit of generosity through acts of kindness and meaningful human connections can trigger a positive chemical response within our bodies, fostering a deeper sense of well-being and satisfaction.

The Impact of Proactive Care

By engaging in proactive conversations and taking charge of our health, we can not only prevent illnesses but also reduce healthcare costs and improve insurance reimbursement. When we invest in preventive care and actively participate in our own well-being, we create a healthier and more sustainable healthcare system for everyone and, most importantly, prolong our lifespan and quality of life.

This book aims to inspire, educate, and empower individuals to take control of their health. By advocating for holistic, proactive care and engaging in meaningful conversations with their doctors, readers will learn to confidently make lifestyle modifications that incorporate a holistic approach considering the whole person. They will also learn to navigate the healthcare system, make informed decisions, and ultimately lead healthier and more fulfilling lives.

In the following chapters, we will explore holistic approaches to preventing the development of diseases and conditions, as well as the maintenance of preexisting health problems. Your Personal Plan of Action will delve into practical strategies for engaging in proactive conversations with your doctor, making informed choices about your health, and taking ownership of your well-being. By the end of this book, you will have the tools and inspiration to venture on a journey toward proactive care and empowered health.

Holistic Journey

Are you ready to embark on a journey towards holistic wellness? Throughout this book, we will explore various aspects of health and well-being, offering practical tips and valuable insights to help you thrive. Have you ever considered alternatives to medication or surgery, or pondered how you reached this point? These questions often go unanswered, but the goal of this book is to shed light on preventive measures that can guide you through each day. The way we start our day significantly impacts our well-being and influences how we approach life's challenges. Our thoughts play a crucial role in shaping our spiritual and emotional well-being. Positive thinking can fill us with energy, while negativity can leave us drained. Let's nurture positivity and embrace hope for a brighter future. It's time to let go of fears and anxieties and believe in the power of meditation, breathing, and relaxation. We will delve deeper into emotional and spiritual well-being soon, but for now, let's begin by discussing the importance of nutrition, as a nourishing breakfast sets the stage for a fulfilling day.

2.
FUELING YOUR WELLNESS: THE POWER OF NUTRITION

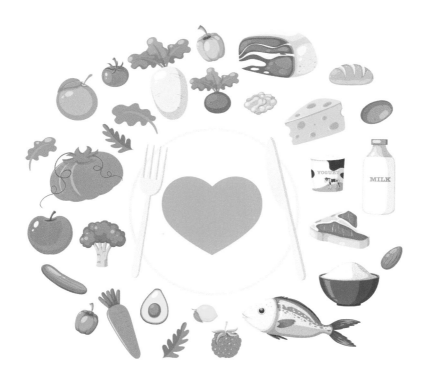

On our journey towards a healthier lifestyle, grasping the importance of the six vital nutrients is crucial. These nutrients play a significant role in providing energy and maintaining our body's equilibrium. Water tops the list as a crucial element, constituting 40%-60% of our body weight and being indispensable for our well-being. Adequate hydration not only combats tiredness but also prevents dehydration. Health experts advise a daily intake of around 3.5

pints of water. Deficiency in nutrients can disrupt metabolism, tissue function, and repair processes. Essential vitamins and nutrients are necessary for biochemical functions, yet lifestyle choices and health conditions can impede their absorption. To rebalance, consider supplementation, dietary adjustments, and lifestyle modifications.

Carbohydrates play a crucial role in providing fuel and energy to our bodies. It's important never to exclude them, as doing so can lead to a condition called ketosis, where the body uses up its fat storage for fuel and energy. Eat whole grains, like cereals, breads, and pasta, in moderation, and avoid refined foods. These unrefined grains provide energy and help prevent diseases. Fruits and starchy vegetables like carrots, potatoes, and berries fulfill the body's carbohydrate needs.

Protein is essential for building muscle mass, but like all good things, it should be consumed in moderation. Excessive protein intake can lead to health issues such as osteoporosis, kidney failure, heart disease, and cancer, particularly if it comes from a diet high in animal proteins. To strike the right balance, consider including plant-based foods in your diet, as they contain both protein and carbohydrates. Protein undernutrition can lead to stunted growth, anemia, weakness, edema, vascular issues, and weakened immunity. Short-term studies recommend specific protein intake for different activity levels, with long-term consumption guidelines for adults.

Fats are necessary for processing vitamins and minerals and insulating our inner organs. The body's response to deficient or excessive states of these nutrients can contribute to various illnesses and diseases, so it's crucial to tune in to our body's reactions to the foods we eat. Include mono-unsaturated and poly-unsaturated fats in your diet, like olive or canola oil. Limit butter, cream, and animal fats, as they can lead to health issues. Consider fish, salmon, tuna, and flax seed oil, as they contain beneficial Omega-3 and Omega-6, which can help lower bad cholesterol.

Maintaining good health involves supplementing your diet with sufficient amounts of antioxidants, zinc, and a variety of vitamins obtained from foods like kale, spinach, beets, fruits, vegetables, seeds, nuts, beans, organic meats, poultry, and alternatives such as quinoa and sweet potatoes. Incorporating beverages like lemon water or cranberry juice can also promote liver health. Vitamins play a crucial role in the body's functioning. There are two kinds of fats: fat-soluble and water-soluble. Fat-soluble vitamins, including A, D, E, and K, are stored in the body's fat reserves and can accumulate if unused. Water-soluble vitamins like B and C are eliminated from the body daily if there is an excess. It's essential to obtain sufficient vitamins from our diet to maintain good health and prevent illnesses. Some vitamins are not produced in our bodies or are insufficiently produced. For instance, Vitamin A is vital for vision, immune function, and can be found in liver or fish. Vitamin C, present in fruits and vegetables, is essential for bone health, skin, and immune function. Vitamin E, found in leafy greens and whole grains, acts as an antioxidant.

Minerals are needed to help the body's enzymes work. They help make enzymes, hormones, bones, teeth, and body fluids. If there's too little or too much of a mineral, it can cause problems, like heart rhythm issues from low or high potassium levels. Intestinal problems, like leaky gut or diarrhea, can cause us to not get enough minerals.

Take Care of Your Tummy:

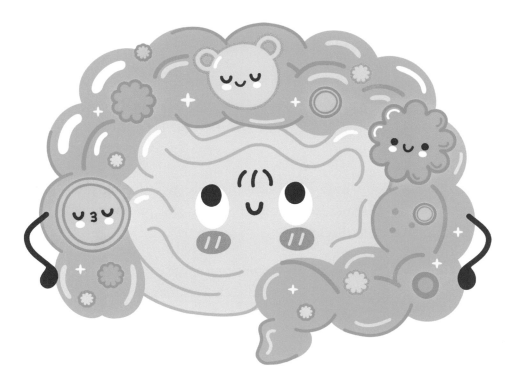

In the journey to achieve optimal gut wellness, it's important to chew your food thoroughly and eat slowly. Swallowing food whole can disrupt the digestion process and lead to digestive issues. It's also important to maintain proper sitting posture during meals by sitting up straight and avoiding lying down after eating, as this can aid in the digestion process.

Healing a "Leaky Gut" often involves an elimination diet, which means temporarily removing specific food groups and gradually reintroducing them while observing the body's response. The goal is to identify and eliminate food groups that trigger adverse reactions in the gut.

Incorporating Omega-3 rich foods can help reduce inflammation and promote overall gut health. Additionally, including glutamine and probiotics in your diet is essential to support intestinal metabolism and optimize the natural flora within the intestinal wall.

A fiber-rich diet is essential for digestive health and regular elimination patterns. Choosing fruits and vegetables that aid regular elimination without causing discomfort is advisable. It's important to consume moderate to small portions of foods such as cabbage, legumes, and apples, as they may induce bloating and gas. While apples are a valuable source of fiber, it's best to consume them in smaller portions and limit intake to once a day.

By incorporating more whole foods like fruits, vegetables, and fiber-rich foods into your diet, you're providing essential nutrients for your body to thrive. Adding antioxidant-rich foods can help combat free radicals and support your overall health.

Taking care of your gut health is crucial as well. Introducing probiotics and prebiotics into your routine can support a healthy gut microbiome, benefiting your immune system and digestion.

Understanding and embracing the significance of these essential nutrients empowers us to make informed and positive choices for our well-being.

Essential Nutrients:

- Vitamin C & D: Supports immune function.
- Omega-3 Fats: Reduces inflammation.
- Zinc: Aids in cell function.
- Probiotics: Maintains gut health.

Healthy Food Choices:

- Proteins: Nuts, seeds, beans, wild fish, organic chicken.
- Carbohydrates: Fresh vegetables, fruits, whole grains.
- Fats: Olive oil, avocado, fish oil.

Eating Habits:

- Eat early and in small portions.
- Focus on balanced meals with a mix of proteins, carbs, and fats.

3.
LET'S ENERGIZE AND GET YOUR BODY MOVING!

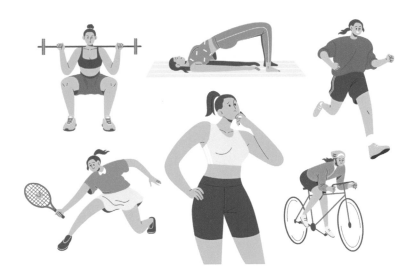

In your wellness journey, remember that exercise and training play a key role in enhancing the function of vital body systems over time. Training allows your body to adapt to exercise and improve athletic performance, in addition to boosting muscle performance and optimizing oxygen delivery to working muscles.

When it comes to physical activity, it's good to focus on endurance and strength. Endurance involves sustaining maximal force repeatedly. Activities like running and cycling can help increase oxygen delivery to the blood and stimulate the production of essential components like hemoglobin. On the other hand, strength training, which includes exercises like weightlifting and jump rope, helps build muscles and improve muscle power. Ensuring adequate protein intake, especially post-workout, is crucial to support muscle growth and strength. Carbohydrates are also essential to fuel your workouts - opt for fruits and vegetables to obtain glucose and consider incorporating berries into your diet as a lower-sugar option.

Moreover, maintaining an adequate oxygen supply is crucial to sustain exercise. Embracing diverse training approaches like resistance and cross-training can help increase your body's oxygen-carrying capacity and enhance cardiac output and respiratory function. Stretching, especially through practices like yoga, not only minimizes muscle soreness and injury but also helps replenish oxygen levels through controlled breathing.

Let's get started and do whatever makes you feel good, is convenient, and aligns with your abilities to commit to the program. You can dance like no one is watching, do squats while washing dishes, or dance around the house. Alternatively, you could revisit the old days and try jumping rope, walking, jogging, or aerobics. You can find some great workout videos on YouTube. It's all about taking small steps to become healthier, happier, and less stressed. Be creative, have fun, don't overthink it, and no excuses. Be consistent with whatever movement you use to get your body and mind back on track or keep you on track. You got this! All you must do is "do it," like Nike.

Remember to pace your exercises and avoid overexertion, which can lead to injuries. It's essential to have a balanced diet with protein and healthy carbohydrates before and after training to support strength and endurance. Resting is also crucial to reduce stress on your body.

Stretching after exercise helps prevent muscle soreness and injury. With stretching and controlled breathing, yoga can be a good option for those who can't do endurance or strength exercises.

Over time, exercise improves the function of your heart, muscles, blood vessels, lungs, nervous system, and skin. It helps your body better respond to exercise and improves athletic performance, muscle function, and oxygen delivery to working muscles.

Embrace the journey to wellness with these principles in mind and keep pushing towards a stronger, healthier you.

Benefits:

- Weight management.
- Stress reduction.
- Improved mental health.
- Enhances Productivity and Concentration
- Reduce the risk of Heart Disease, and Diabetes.
- Improve Digestive system and Immune function

Recommendations:

- Dedicate at least 30 minutes each day to exercise.
- Include a mix of cardio, strength training, and flexibility exercises.

4.
SUFFICIENT REST

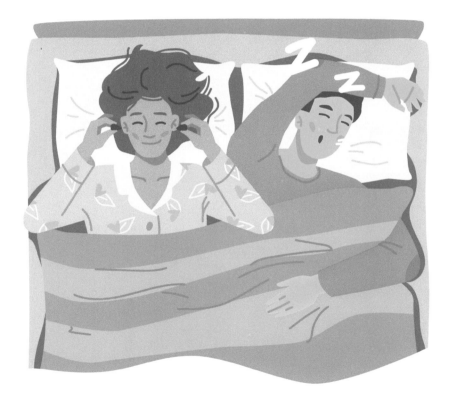

Getting an adequate amount of sleep is vital for maintaining good health. Health experts recommend getting between seven to eight hours of sleep each night, as this is the optimal amount for most adults. However, it's important to acknowledge that some people may find it challenging to reach this goal immediately. In such cases, making progress by starting with at least six hours of sleep is a positive step.

For individuals who struggle with falling asleep, there are various strategies that can be helpful. One option is to consider taking melatonin supplements, a hormone that can aid in regulating the sleep-wake cycle. Another approach is to consume sleepy time tea before bedtime, as the ingredients in this type of tea, such as chamomile, may promote relaxation and ease the transition into sleep.

In addition to these remedies, creating a soothing sleep environment is beneficial. Introducing calming scents, particularly lavender, to your surroundings can contribute to a more restful sleep experience. Lavender has been shown to have relaxing properties, and using lavender-scented products or essential oils in the bedroom may help to promote a sense of tranquility and enhance sleep quality.

Importance:

- Rest is crucial for physical and mental recovery.
- Adequate sleep supports immune function and cognitive performance.

Tips:

- Aim for 7-9 hours of sleep per night.
- Maintain a consistent sleep schedule.
- Create a restful sleeping environment.

5.
MINIMIZING EXPOSURE TO ENVIRONMENTAL TOXINS

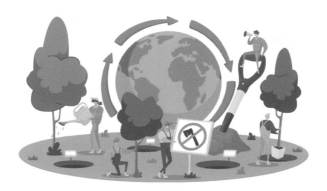

When it comes to improving your environment for your well-being, you can consider introducing a variety of elements such as vibrant colors, calming scents, pleasant aromas, soothing sounds, and captivating scenery. Ensuring that you eliminate any toxins or allergens from your surroundings is crucial, as these substances have been shown to disrupt the functioning of your immune system. Inhaling toxic agents or allergens can lead to inflammation in the body, which can have wide-ranging effects on your health. It's vital to be vigilant about protecting your environment from negative energy. Take the time to identify and remove any sources of negativity, no matter how challenging it may seem. Conducting a thorough inventory of your surroundings can be highly beneficial in uncovering elements that may be contributing to illness and impacting your overall state of wellness.

Common Toxins:

- Metals (mercury, lead, arsenic).
- Pesticides and industrial chemicals.
- Toxins in food, cleaning supplies, and containers.

Strategies:

- Opt for organic produce.
- Use natural cleaning products.
- Avoid processed foods and excessive alcohol/tobacco use.

6.
EXPLORING SPIRITUALITY AND WELLNESS FOR GOOD HEALTH AND WELL-BEING

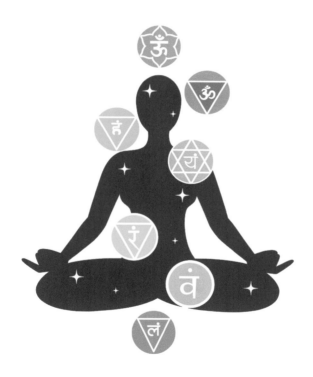

n our life journey, it's important to explore our personal spirituality and our worldview and shift our focus from illness to health. Prioritizing activities that bring us joy can help us see life, health, and illness as a gift. This change in perspective can lead to a profound sense of joy and a greater appreciation for life, allowing us to overcome any situation, especially when it comes to our health and unexpected health conditions and diagnosis. It's essential to look for opportunities to fill our days with a renewed sense of purpose and accomplishment. Prayer can offer the support and strength to pull through and achieve our health and wellness goals.

Let's not ignore the messages our bodies are sending us. By increasing our self-awareness, we come to understand that our health is far more within our control than we might have previously believed. Taking an active role in our well-being, making positive lifestyle changes, and striving for balance and wellness enable us to release the sole responsibility of restoring health from our doctors and embark on a journey of proactive self-care and empowerment.

Thriving in Good Health and Well-Being

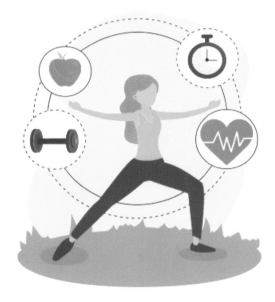

Maintaining overall wellness involves prioritizing your physical well-being through healthy eating, regular exercise, and enjoyable activities. It's also important to focus on positive thinking by avoiding negativity, practicing relaxation techniques like meditation and controlled breathing, and surrounding yourself with uplifting influences. Additionally, expressing yourself openly, nurturing meaningful connections, and being mindful of your surroundings all contribute to your overall wellness. Take care of your physical, psychological, and spiritual well-being to achieve inner balance and fulfillment.

Tips for Optimal Health:

- Eat early and in small portions.
- Prioritize regular exercise, even if it's just 15-30 minutes a day.
- Manage stress, as it can impact sugar levels, insulin resistance, elevate blood pressure, and impair immune function.
- Engage in meaningful activities, be creative, find your purpose, practice gratitude, exercise, and limit caffeine intake for a calmer mind and body.

Key Elements:

- Nutrition: Balanced diet with essential nutrients.
- Exercise: Regular physical activity.
- Stress Management: Techniques like meditation and relaxation.

Additional Factors:

- Adequate water intake.
- Exposure to natural light and fresh air.
- Cultivating love and a balanced routine.
- Even if you're not experiencing physical symptoms, feelings of boredom, depression, tension, anxiety, or unhappiness can lead to stress and potential health issues.

Identifying and Eliminating Excess

Are there elements in your life or environment that are in abundance and need to be eliminated?

In both cases, toxins, allergens, and microbes can be overwhelming. For instance, mental, emotional, and spiritual toxins should be eliminated, as well as heavy metals like mercury, lead, and arsenic, internal toxins such as bacteria and mold, and toxic foods like sugar and trans fats.

Cultivating a Spirit of Generosity

Benefits:

- Acts of kindness trigger positive chemical responses.
- Enhances satisfaction and well-being.

Tips:

- Volunteer in your community.
- Practice daily acts of kindness.
- Build and maintain meaningful human connections.

7.
FACTORS CONTRIBUTING TO ILLNESS

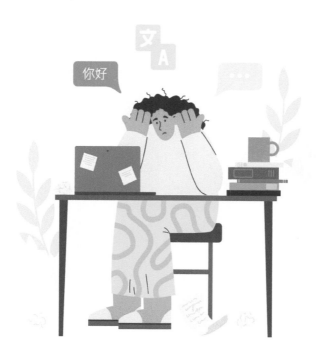

To understand the underlying reasons for illness and imbalance, we need to look beyond surface-level symptoms. Although it's easy to see the effects of illness and health, the factors that influence our lifestyle choices are deeper and more complex. By examining our values and environment, we can uncover their impact on our overall health, which can help us lead a more meaningful and balanced life. Let's explore further and uncover what lies beneath the surface.

The environment around us can greatly affect our well-being. Negative energy in our surroundings can lead to overeating, substance abuse, and poor healing. Remember, stress weakens the immune system, making us more prone to illness and delaying recovery.

Predisposing Factors:

- Genetics: Inherited traits.
- Lifestyle: Diet, exercise, and habits.
- Environment: Toxins, stressors, and trauma.

Illness Contributors:

- Absence of affection, human interaction and individual satisfaction.
- Prolonged stress can have a significant impact on both physical and mental health.
- Environmental toxins, pollutants, stressors, and allergens.
- Negative psychosocial experiences.
- Poor diet and lack of exercise.

The Impact of Nutrition on Handling Stress

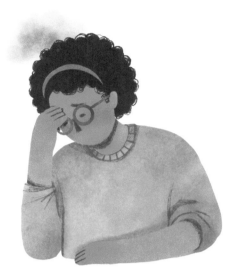

Have you ever considered the effect of what you eat on how your body deals with stress? Research has shown that during times of prolonged stress, certain nutrients play a vital role in supporting our bodies. These include protein, vitamin B complex, vitamins A, C, and E, unsaturated fatty acids, minerals, and cholesterol. These nutrients help our adrenal glands produce corticosteroids, assisting our bodies in coping with ongoing stress and maintaining balance.

Prolonged stress can lead to habits like overeating, particularly for those who turn to comfort foods. This can result in weight gain and impact our mood. Instead of reaching for high-calorie and fatty foods, consider incorporating nuts into your diet as they are rich in essential nutrients like protein, fiber, and various vitamins and minerals. Additionally, deficiencies in essential nutrients like zinc and vitamin B can lead to symptoms such as fatigue, attention deficit, and weakness.

To support your body during stressful times, consider increasing your intake of certain nutrients and incorporating healthier food choices. Supplementing with vitamin C and consuming foods rich in fatty acids also plays a role in managing stress. By paying attention to what we eat, we can better support our bodies in handling stress and maintaining overall well-being.

Understanding Our Body

Our body can get sick from things in our environment, like the food we eat and the air we breathe. Things like stress and not eating well can also make us sick.

Staying Strong and Balanced:

- Eat healthy a balanced meal
- Exercise regularly.
- Ensure our body's systems are working properly with Lifestyle modifications.

Herbs/Tea blends for Stress and Adrenal Function

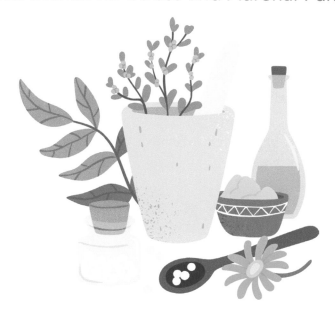

Ashwagandha

Use- Adaptogen, used for adrenal function and counteract the biological changes accompanying severe stress, including changes in blood sugar and cortisol levels.

Dosage- 2- 3 g twice daily

Contraindication - well tolerated but can cause GI intolerance in high dosages.

Holy basil

Use - Helps with metabolic health, including regulating blood glucose, cholesterol, blood pressure, insomnia, and antioxidants.

Indication - Stress, insomnia,

Rhodiola

Use - Adaptogen influences neurotransmitters serotonin, dopamine, and norepinephrine levels and protects against oxidative stress (reduces inflammation in the neurological system) and fatigue.
Indication- Modulates stress response, depression, cardioprotective, anti-inflammatory, and physical performance.
Dosage - 100- 300mg three times a day.
Contraindication: Studies show interaction with some medications, including anti-depressants.
Side Effects - Can cause dry mouth and dizziness.

Licorice (Dried Root, demulcent)

Use - Inflammation, Liver conditions, respiratory issues
Indication - effects on the endocrine system and liver-
Contraindication- Should not be used for individuals using diuretics and antihypertensive agents.
Side Effects -Hypertension, headache, salt retention, hypokalemia,
Dosage - 1-4g daily TID

Lemon Balm (Capsule of dried leaf or tincture)

Use - promote sleep, aromatherapy (Uplifting energy)
Indication -Insomnia
Dosage - 300mg -500mg or 60 drops
Contraindication - should not be used by pregnant or lactating women.

L-Theanine (amino acid found in green or black tea)

Use - Insomnia

Indication - Managing anxiety, Hypertension, sleeplessness,

Dosage - 50- 400mg taken 30- 60 minutes before bedtime.

Contraindication - not recommended for pregnant or lactating women; antihypertensive effects should be used with caution and under the physician's supervision if taking antihypertensive medications.

B-Complex

Protects adrenal function, decreases the stress-induced cortisol response, supports sleep quality, and are essential cofactors necessary to produce neurotransmitters (important for optimal neurological functioning)

Vitamin B6

B6 (Pyridoxine) (Pyridoxal Phosphate) - deficiency is linked to mood and psychological disturbance.

8.
THE MIND-BODY CONNECTION

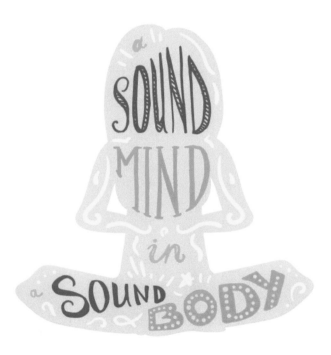

We are like energy transformers connected to the universe. How we manage our energy impacts our health and well-being. Humans take in energy, transform it, and release it back into the environment. The smooth flow of energy is essential for our overall well-being. Each of us is a unique channel of energy, affecting how much energy we absorb and radiate. We feel good when the energy flow is harmonious, but feel disoriented when there's interference. We need to ensure proper air circulation, access to nutritious food, and opportunities for social connection and love. Along with physical stimuli, emotional and spiritual inputs like attention, compassion, love, and enthusiasm are crucial. It's important to pay attention to our emotions, thoughts, intuition, dreams, and spiritual insights.

Impact:

- Mental states can influence physical health.
- Positive thoughts and emotions contribute to well-being.

Strategies for Relaxation and Well-Being

The relaxation response is a state of deep rest that can be achieved through various methods, such as meditation, yoga, and progressive muscle relaxation. These techniques are proven to be effective in reducing stress and improving our response to it. Writing down our thoughts and emotions or letting them out through writing can be quite effective in contrast to keeping them inside. Other common techniques include:

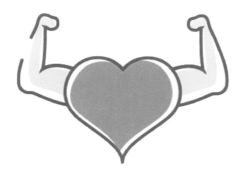

- Progressive Muscle Relaxation: This involves slowly tensing and relaxing each muscle group to increase awareness of physical sensations. You can start by tensing and then relaxing your muscles from either the head down or the feet up. Tighten your muscles for 5 seconds, then relax for 30 seconds, and repeat.

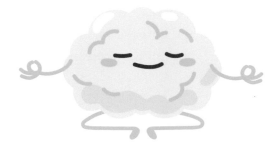

- Mindfulness Meditation: Begin by using concentration meditation to find calmness and stability, followed by focusing on observation. When thoughts or feelings arise, don't push them aside or judge them. Instead, observe each thought without judgment, allowing you to see things clearly and accept them as they are in the moment.

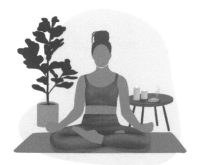

- Yoga: Yoga is a holistic practice involving physical, mental, and spiritual development. Through positions and exercises, it promotes physical and mental harmony, healing, and strength. It can also reduce muscle tension and prepare the body for mental relaxation. Tai chi and Qigong involve slow, gentle movements, deep breathing, and meditation techniques to foster wellness and a calm mind.

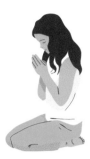

- Repetitive Prayer: Engaging in prayer or meditation while focusing on regular breathing and silently repeating a Bible verse or short phrase can help the mind focus and find inner calm.

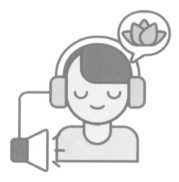

- Guided Imagery: This technique aids in visualizing oneself in a desired state, helping to reduce anxiety and improve coping skills.

By practicing these techniques, you can effectively manage stress and cultivate a sense of well-being and inner peace.

9.
ESTABLISHING AND PURSUING SIGNIFICANT GOALS, PURPOSE, AND ACHIEVING BALANCE

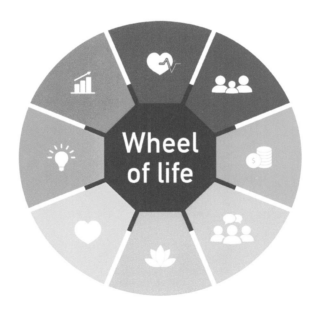

The wellness wheel is a helpful tool that enables us to identify areas in our lives that require attention, care, and modification. It's essential to make time for activities that bring us joy, laughter, and intimacy, even if that means spending time alone to learn and develop ourselves. Practicing self-love and intimacy is crucial to our overall well-being and happiness.

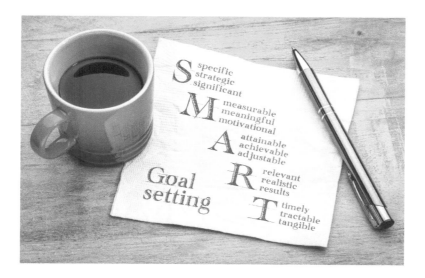

Changing our health behaviors can be a daunting task for many of us, but fear not, for there are numerous strategies we can employ to make this journey easier. One powerful strategy is goal setting, which allows us to pinpoint the specific behaviors we want to change and outline the steps to make this change a reality. However, setting a goal is just the beginning. Sometimes, finding the right goal can be a challenge, and putting that goal into action can be even more difficult. That's where our two powerful strategies come into play. First, by understanding the characteristics of our goals, such as approach vs. avoidance goals, performance vs. mastery goals, and level of difficulty, we can select goals that are appropriate and achievable. Second, through action planning, we can turn our goals into actionable steps, paving the way for success. Embracing these strategies can lead us toward a path of transformation and empowerment, helping us not only set meaningful goals but also achieve them.

Benefits:

- Enhances overall well-being.
- Provides a sense of accomplishment.

Tips:

- Choose work that aligns with your values and passions.
- Set and pursue meaningful career goals.

Impact:

- Helps achieve a sense of purpose.
- Boosts motivation and personal growth.

Strategies:

- Set SMART goals (Specific, Measurable, Achievable, Relevant, Time-bound).
- Regularly review and adjust your goals.

10.
THRIVING THROUGH ACTION: VITAL TIPS FOR PARTICIPATION AND WELLNESS

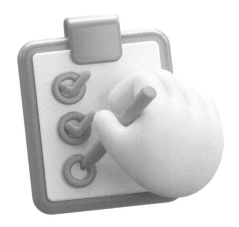

1. Be an Active Participant:
   ○ Take charge of your healthcare decisions.

2. Ask Questions:
   ○ Be inquisitive about your health and treatments.

3. Change Attitudes:
   ○ Adopt a positive outlook towards health.

4. Learn Coping Skills:
   ○ Develop strategies to handle stress.

5. Maintain Humor:
   - Find joy and laughter in everyday moments.

6. Use Love as a Healing Tool:
   - Foster loving relationships.

7. Choose Happiness:
   - opt for positivity in life.

8. Responsibility:
   - Be accountable for your choices and actions.

9. Intimate Relationships:
   - Build deep connections with others.

10. Express Affection:
    - Physical touch can enhance relaxation.

11. Laughter:
    - Promotes a healthy immune function.

12. Manage Anger:
    - Use techniques like deep breathing and communication.

13. Learn to Say "No":
    - Protect your well-being by setting boundaries.

14. Control Life Choices:
    - Make informed and thoughtful decisions.

15. Engage in Creativity:
    - Use art and music for stress relief.

16. Nourish Your Body:
    - Balance action, diet, relaxation, and spirituality.

17. Make Time to Play:
    - Engage in fun activities.

18. Express Yourself:
    - Find healthy outlets for your thoughts and emotions.

19. Enjoy Life Moments:
    - Embrace life's experiences, even during illness.

Wellness Reflections: Assessing Your Path to Wholeness

Complete this section to evaluate your current wellness status.

Physical Health

- How would you describe your current level of physical activity? What changes, if any, would you like to make?
- How do your eating habits contribute to your overall energy and vitality?
- What steps can you take to improve your sleep quality?

Emotional Wellness

- How do you typically manage stress? Are there more effective strategies you could try?
- What emotions do you experience most often, and how do they impact your daily life?
- How do you express your emotions? What areas could you work on to improve emotional balance?

Intellectual Wellness

- What activities challenge your mind and stimulate your curiosity?
- How do you continue learning and expanding your knowledge?
- What new skills or hobbies would you like to develop?

Social Wellness

- How would you describe the quality of your relationships with family, friends, and colleagues?
- In what ways do you support and nurture your social connections?
- How do you balance time spent alone with time spent with others?

Spiritual Wellness

- What gives your life meaning and purpose? How do you connect with this regularly?
- How do you practice gratitude or mindfulness in your daily life?
- In what ways do you seek to connect with something larger than yourself?

Environmental Wellness

- How do your surroundings affect your mood and well-being?
- What steps can you take to create a healthier and more supportive environment?
- How do you engage with and care for the natural world around you?

Occupational Wellness

- How satisfied are you with your current work or daily activities?
- What aspects of your work bring you the most fulfillment?
- How do you maintain a healthy work-life balance?

Financial Wellness

- How do you feel about your current financial situation?
- What steps can you take to improve your financial security?
- How do you manage stress related to money?

Mental Wellness

- What practices help you maintain mental clarity and focus?
- How do you manage negative thought patterns or cognitive distortions?
- What role does mental health play in your overall well-being, and how do you support it?

Creative Wellness

- How do you express yourself creatively?
- What activities allow you to explore your imagination and creativity?
- How does engaging in creative pursuits enhance your overall sense of well-being?

Personal Growth and Development

- What goals are you currently working toward? How do they align with your values and passions?
- What habits or routines support your personal growth?
- How do you reflect on your progress and celebrate your achievements?

Life Purpose and Fulfillment

- What do you feel is your life's purpose, and how do you align your actions with this purpose?
- How do you define fulfillment, and what steps can you take to achieve it?
- What legacy do you wish to leave behind, and how are you working toward it?

Stress Management

- What are your current stressors, and how are they affecting your well-being?
- What techniques do you use to manage and reduce stress?
- How can you incorporate more relaxation and mindfulness into your daily routine?

Time Management

- How effectively do you manage your time, and what areas could be improved?
- What priorities guide how you spend your time each day?
- How do you ensure that you make time for self-care and relaxation?

Healthy Relationships

- What qualities do you value most in your relationships?
- How do you maintain healthy boundaries in your interactions with others?
- What steps can you take to improve communication and connection in your relationships?

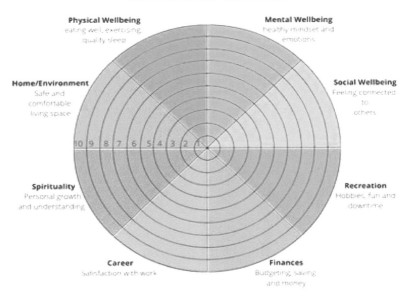

Wellness Wheel

Retrieved from https://www.vibrantsoulful.com/post/how-to-use-a-wellness-wheel

Self-Assessment Score:

- Physical Health: ___ / 10
- Nutrition: ___ / 10
- Mental Health: ___ / 10
- Sleep: ___ / 10
- Relationships: ___ / 10
- Finances: ___ /10
- Career: ___/10
- Spirituality: ___ / 10

Self-Assessment Score: _____

Defining Wellness Objectives

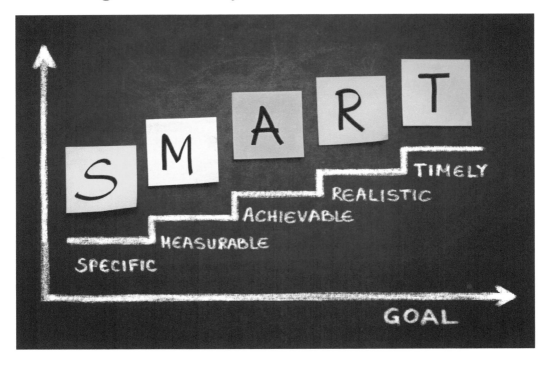

Set clear and achievable wellness goals. Use the SMART criteria (Specific, Measurable, Attainable, Relevant, Time-bound).

Example Objectives:

1. Physical Health: Walk 10,000 steps daily for the next month.
2. Nutrition: Incorporate at least 5 servings of fruits and vegetables into daily meals.
3. Mental Health: Practice mindfulness meditation for 10 minutes every day.
4. Sleep: Aim for 7-8 hours of sleep each night.
5. Relationships: Schedule weekly catchups with friends or family.

Wellness Goals and Action Steps

Outline your wellness goals and the steps needed to achieve them.

Goal 1:

- Objective: _____
- Action Steps:

_____

_____

_____

Goal 2:

- Objective: _____
- Action Steps:

_____

_____

_____

Goal 3:

- Objective: _____
- Action Steps:

_____

_____

_____

Goal 4:

- Objective: _____
- Action Steps:

_____

_____

_____

Goal 5:

- Objective: _____
- Action Steps:

_____

_____

_____

Goal 6:

- Objective: _____
- Action Steps:

_____

_____

_____

Goal 7:

- Objective: _____
- Action Steps:

_____

_____

_____

Goal 8:

- Objective: _____
- Action Steps:

_____

_____

_____

Goal 9:

- Objective: _____
- Action Steps:

_____

_____

_____

Goal 10:

- Objective: _____
- Action Steps:

_____

_____

_____

Mindfulness Practices

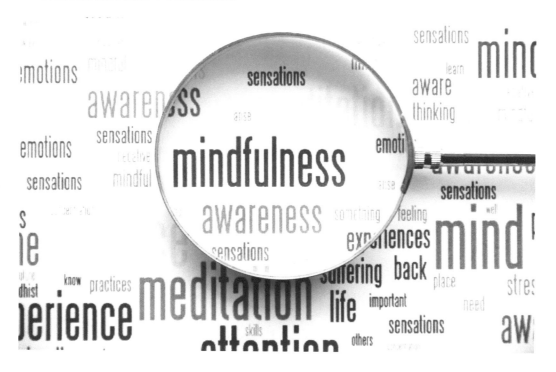

Integrate mindfulness techniques to improve mental and emotional wellness.

Consider these insightful questions to help navigate and enrich your mindfulness practice.

1. Body Awareness

Instruction: Find a comfortable position, sitting or lying down. Close your eyes and take a few deep breaths. Start scanning your body from head to toe, noticing any areas of tension or discomfort. Breathe into these areas, observing how they feel without trying to change them. Gradually work your way through your entire body, bringing your full attention to each part.

- What physical sensations do you notice in your body right now?
- Can you locate any tension in your body? What happens when you breathe into that area?
- How does your body feel when you focus on a specific part, like your hands or feet?

2. Mindful Breathing

Instruction: Sit or lie down in a comfortable position. Close your eyes and bring your attention to your breath. Notice the sensation of the air as it enters through your nose, fills your lungs, and exits through your mouth or nose. If your mind wanders, gently bring your focus back to your breath. Continue this for a few minutes, simply observing your breath without trying to control it.

- How does your breath feel as it enters and leaves your body?
- What happens to your thoughts and emotions when you focus solely on your breath?
- Can you notice the slight pause between your inhale and exhale? How does this make you feel?

3. Emotional Awareness

Instruction: Sit quietly and take a few deep breaths to center yourself. Notice what emotions you are feeling at this moment. Try to identify and name them without judgment. Observe where you feel these emotions in your body. Allow yourself to experience them fully without trying to change or suppress them.

- What emotions are you experiencing right now? Can you name them?
- How does your body react to different emotions?
- What happens when you observe your emotions without trying to change them?

4. Mindful Listening

Instruction: Sit comfortably and close your eyes. Begin to focus on the sounds around you. Notice both near and distant sounds and observe how they come and go. Try not to judge or label the sounds; simply listen to them as they are. If thoughts distract you, gently return your attention to listening.

- What sounds do you notice around you when you sit quietly?
- How does it feel to listen to someone without interrupting or planning your response?
- What do you notice about the quality of different sounds?

5. Gratitude Practice

Instruction: Take a moment to reflect on three things you are grateful for today. These can be big or small, significant or simple. Write them down or say them aloud. Focus on the feelings of gratitude that arise as you think about each one and allow yourself to fully experience those feelings.

- What are three things you are grateful for at this moment?
- How does focusing on gratitude change your mood or perspective?
- What small thing happened today that you can appreciate?

6. Present Moment Awareness

Instruction: Wherever you are, take a moment to pause and notice your surroundings. Pay attention to what you see, hear, smell, taste, and feel. Focus on each of your senses in turn, fully immersing yourself in the present moment. If your mind drifts, gently guide it back to the sensations of the here and now.

- What is happening right now, in this moment? What can you see, hear, feel, smell, or taste?
- How does focusing on the present moment affect your thoughts and emotions?
- What thoughts pull you away from the present moment, and how do you bring yourself back?

7. Mindful Eating

Instruction: Choose a piece of food to eat slowly and mindfully. Before eating, observe the food's color, texture, and smell. Take a small bite and notice how it feels in your mouth, how it tastes, and how your body responds as you chew and swallow. Eat slowly, savoring each bite and staying fully present in the experience.

- How does your food taste when you eat it slowly and mindfully?
- What sensations do you notice in your mouth and body as you eat?
- How does paying attention to your eating habits change your experience of food?

8. Mindful Walking

Instruction: As you walk, slow your pace and focus on the sensations in your body. Notice how your feet feel as they touch the ground, how your muscles engage with each step, and how your breath synchronizes with your movements. Pay attention to your surroundings, observing the sights, sounds, and smells with curiosity and openness.

- What do you notice about your surroundings when you walk slowly and mindfully?
- How does your body feel as you take each step?
- How does walking mindfully affect your thoughts and emotions?

9. Compassion Practice

Instruction: Sit quietly and recall someone who you care about, including yourself. Silently repeat phrases like "May you be happy, may you be healthy, may you be safe, may you live with ease." Focus on sending feelings of warmth and kindness to this person. You can also extend this compassion to others, including people you have conflicts with.

- What happens when you send kind thoughts to yourself and others?
- How does it feel to practice self-compassion in difficult moments?
- Can you observe how compassion impacts your interactions with others?

10. Mindful Reflection

Instruction: At the end of your mindfulness practice or day, take a few minutes to reflect on your experiences. Consider what you learned about yourself, how you felt during the practice, and how it has impacted your overall well-being. Write down your thoughts or simply sit with them, allowing the insights to deepen.

- What did you learn about yourself through this mindfulness practice?
- How has your understanding of mindfulness changed after engaging in these activities?
- What challenges did you face, and how did you overcome them?

Daily Mindfulness Log:

- Date: _____
- Practice Duration: _____ minutes
- Technique Used: _____
- Reflections: _____

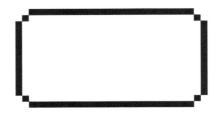

Daily Mindfulness Log:

- Date: _____
- Practice Duration: _____ minutes
- Technique Used: _____
- Reflections: _____

Daily Mindfulness Log:

- Date: _____
- Practice Duration: _____ minutes
- Technique Used: _____
- Reflections: _____

Daily Mindfulness Log:

- Date: _____
- Practice Duration: _____ minutes
- Technique Used: _____
- Reflections: _____

Daily Mindfulness Log:

- Date: _____
- Practice Duration: _____ minutes
- Technique Used: _____
- Reflections: _____

Daily Mindfulness Log:

- Date: _____
- Practice Duration: _____ minutes
- Technique Used: _____
- Reflections: _____

Daily Mindfulness Log:

- Date: _____
- Practice Duration: _____ minutes
- Technique Used: _____
- Reflections: _____

Daily Mindfulness Log:

- Date: _____
- Practice Duration: _____ minutes
- Technique Used: _____
- Reflections: _____

Daily Mindfulness Log:

- Date: _____
- Practice Duration: _____ minutes
- Technique Used: _____
- Reflections: _____

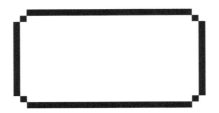

Daily Mindfulness Log:

- Date: _____
- Practice Duration: _____ minutes
- Technique Used: _____
- Reflections: _____

Daily Mindfulness Log:

- Date: _____
- Practice Duration: _____ minutes
- Technique Used: _____
- Reflections: _____

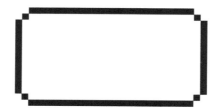

Daily Mindfulness Log:

- Date: _____
- Practice Duration: _____ minutes
- Technique Used: _____
- Reflections: _____

Daily Mindfulness Log:

- Date: _____
- Practice Duration: _____ minutes
- Technique Used: _____
- Reflections: _____

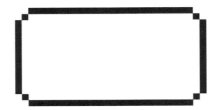

Daily Mindfulness Log:

- Date: _____
- Practice Duration: _____ minutes
- Technique Used: _____
- Reflections: _____

Daily Mindfulness Log:

- Date: _____
- Practice Duration: _____ minutes
- Technique Used: _____
- Reflections: _____

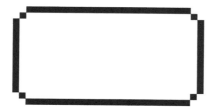

Daily Mindfulness Log:

- Date: _____
- Practice Duration: _____ minutes
- Technique Used: _____
- Reflections: _____

Daily Mindfulness Log:

- Date: _____
- Practice Duration: _____ minutes
- Technique Used: _____
- Reflections: _____

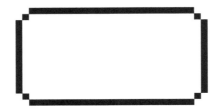

Daily Mindfulness Log:

- Date: _____
- Practice Duration: _____ minutes
- Technique Used: _____
- Reflections: _____

Daily Mindfulness Log:

- Date: _____
- Practice Duration: _____ minutes
- Technique Used: _____
- Reflections: _____

Daily Mindfulness Log:

- Date: _____
- Practice Duration: _____ minutes
- Technique Used: _____
- Reflections: _____

Daily Mindfulness Log:

- Date: _____
- Practice Duration: _____ minutes
- Technique Used: _____
- Reflections: _____

Daily Mindfulness Log:

- Date: _____
- Practice Duration: _____ minutes
- Technique Used: _____
- Reflections: _____

Daily Mindfulness Log:

- Date: _____
- Practice Duration: _____ minutes
- Technique Used: _____
- Reflections: _____

Daily Mindfulness Log:

- Date: _____
- Practice Duration: _____ minutes
- Technique Used: _____
- Reflections: _____

Daily Mindfulness Log:

- Date: _____
- Practice Duration: _____ minutes
- Technique Used: _____
- Reflections: _____

Daily Mindfulness Log:

- Date: _____
- Practice Duration: _____ minutes
- Technique Used: _____
- Reflections: _____

Daily Mindfulness Log:

- Date: _____
- Practice Duration: _____ minutes
- Technique Used: _____
- Reflections: _____

Daily Mindfulness Log:

- Date: _____
- Practice Duration: _____ minutes
- Technique Used: _____
- Reflections: _____

Daily Mindfulness Log:

- Date: _____
- Practice Duration: _____ minutes
- Technique Used: _____
- Reflections: _____

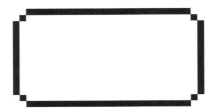

Daily Mindfulness Log:

- Date: _____
- Practice Duration: _____ minutes
- Technique Used: _____
- Reflections: _____

Wholesome Lifestyle

A comprehensive approach to a wholesome lifestyle includes balanced nutrition, regular physical activity, mental and emotional well-being, and consistent health monitoring.

Physical Activity Log

Record your daily physical activities.

Date	Activity	Duration	Intensity	Notes

Nutrition Diary and Journal

Individuals should also be mindful of common food allergy triggers such as milk, wheat, sugar, yeast, and corn. Symptoms associated with food sensitivities can include headaches, coughing, blurred vision, rapid heartbeat, indigestion, skin rashes, fatigue, joint swelling, and mood swings.

For those with a gluten allergy, a gluten-free diet often includes natural and unprocessed beans, seeds, nuts, fresh eggs, meats, fish, poultry, fruits, and vegetables. Additionally, organic and hormone-free dairy products or soy can be suitable alternatives, and for those without allergies to honey, it can be an ideal substitute for sugar.

Keep track of your daily food intake and reflect on your nutritional habits.

Date	Meal	Food Items	Portion Size	Notes

Date	Meal	Food Items	Portion Size	Notes

Date	Meal	Food Items	Portion Size	Notes

Date	Meal	Food Items	Portion Size	Notes

Date	Meal	Food Items	Portion Size	Notes

Date	Meal	Food Items	Portion Size	Notes

Date	Meal	Food Items	Portion Size	Notes

Date	Meal	Food Items	Portion Size	Notes

Date	Meal	Food Items	Portion Size	Notes

Date	Meal	Food Items	Portion Size	Notes

Date	Meal	Food Items	Portion Size	Notes

Date	Meal	Food Items	Portion Size	Notes

Date	Meal	Food Items	Portion Size	Notes

Date	Meal	Food Items	Portion Size	Notes

Date	Meal	Food Items	Portion Size	Notes

Vital Sign Log

Please take note of the following guidelines:

Monitor and record your vital signs regularly.

If your blood pressure falls below 90/50 (especially if you're taking blood pressure medication and experiencing symptoms like lightheadedness, dizziness, fatigue, drowsiness, or feeling unlike yourself) or exceeds 150/100 with symptoms such as headache, blurred vision, chest pain, and heaviness, contact your doctor immediately or seek urgent care or emergency room assistance.

Alert: Maintain a serum glucose level lower than 150 and an HgbA1c level lower than 5.6. Elevated HgbA1c indicates potential diabetes. Consider adjusting your diet to align with a reduced calorie diet, increase physical activity, manage stress, and consult with your doctor for further guidance.

Alert: Keep triglyceride levels below 110, total cholesterol below 220, and HDL (good cholesterol) above 55. Low HDL levels increase the risk of heart disease. Request a lab report to monitor your baseline and make dietary and lifestyle adjustments. Regular exercise and a diet rich in fiber, fruits, vegetables, and Omega-3 can help manage cholesterol levels.

Alert: Maintain a blood pressure below 120/80. Factors such as high salt intake, stress, and lack of physical activity can contribute to elevated blood pressure. Monitor your blood pressure regularly, practice stress-reducing activities like meditation or yoga, and ensure an adequate amount of rest. Consider adjusting your diet to align with the DASH or Mediterranean diet.

Supplements to help address cardiovascular status and normalize lipid panels include garlic, vitamin D, omega-3 fatty acids, vitamin E, flaxseed, vitamin B6, B12, and folate.

Remember that you are in control of your health journey. Keep track of your health, communicate with your healthcare providers, and manage your medications, nutrition, activity levels, and vital signs diligently.

Date	Blood Pressure	Heart Rate	Blood Sugar	Weight	Notes

Physician List with Office Visit Notes

Maintain a record of your healthcare providers and notes from your visits.

Provider Name	Specialty	Contact Information	Last Visit Date	Notes

Medication and Supplement List

Keep track of your medications and supplements.

Medication/ Supplement	Dosage	Frequency	Purpose	Prescribing Doctor	Notes

11.
CONCLUSION

Life is a journey with ups and downs. Embrace every experience, and actively participate in your health and well-being. By following the guidelines in this booklet, you can lead a healthier, more fulfilling life.

Remember, maintaining good health and wellness is an ongoing process. Stay informed, stay active, and stay positive!

This book is intended to provide comprehensive wellness information and does not replace professional medical advice.

Final Tips to Consider:

In our journey for optimal health, it's essential to nourish our bodies with the right foods and supplements. Here are some key points to remember:

1. Green tea EGCG, Milk Thistle, Olive oil, nuts, garlic, pomegranate, and flaxseed all offer unique health benefits, from reducing inflammation to supporting heart and liver health.

2. Supplements such as Omega-3 FA, Vitamin D, Vitamin B complex, and probiotics can play a crucial role in addressing cardiovascular health and normalizing lipid levels.

3. Nutrient deficiencies can disrupt our body's natural processes. Lifestyle factors and health conditions can deplete essential nutrients. This is

       where dietary changes and targeted supplementation come into play to restore balance.

4.   Lastly, maintaining awareness of our alcohol consumption and adjusting it as needed can positively impact our overall health.

Remember, small but consistent changes in our diet and lifestyle can lead to significant improvements in our well-being.

"Something Extra: Poetry Corner"

Journaling and writing poetry have been my way of releasing the thoughts and emotions that are swirling inside me. It has been my most effective medicine and therapy, helping me heal from depression after the sudden death of my father and other life challenges. I hope you can find your own way to release and heal from whatever you are going through, or to help you cope with the everyday hustle of life.

Shattered

The glass shattered on a rainy morning, not knowing
your bones were broken the evening before!

The week before, we rode out on one of our regular road trips to Maryland!

What an incredible ride full of laughs, disagreements,
quietness, and, most importantly, love!

There is nothing like a bond between a daughter and a father!

A bond to cherish until we meet again!

Until then, I will remember you carrying me on your
shoulders as we marched on Eastern Parkway!

I will remember your jokes, sarcasm, craziness, and all the things
and qualities that made you the best father for me!

You taught me how to be reliable, confident, and smart beyond the books!

You shared undeniable wisdom and strength, which
are highly valuable and non-tangible.

Your sudden departure left me shattered, but it's time to mend the
broken pieces, and no longer drown in my sorrow and pain.

I will make you proud and carry on with your plans left undone.

I'm learning to live again and laugh whenever I think of you!

I no longer cry about missing you because I know
your spirit walks with me daily.

I know you will always have my back and be the
warmth I feel over my shoulders!

Love You, Daddy!

Depression

Depression and sadness suck all the joy and visions from
your soul and leave you in a place of darkness.

You become unrecognizable when you face yourself in the mirror.

Your hair is a mess, entangled in knots, causing
you to lose a few inches of your hair.

Followed by that foul smell steaming from your armpits.

Looking around to blame someone for this awful scent,
but it's only you in this dark and stench place.

Entangled in knots, and the scent is keeping no one near!

Your mind is consumed with negative thoughts of
the past, present, and the grim future.

You are hoping for someone to see you or call for you, but you
are lost in darkness and nowhere to be found or heard.

It's just you and your thoughts in this lonely place.

You drift off in your thoughts of how did I let myself get this far, to a
place where no one can recognize me or not even I know who I am.

How long can I stay in this state?

I have so many things to do, places to go, and a life to live, but the light
is dim in this dark place, and it makes it hard to find my way out.

You start to pray and meditate with hopes of finding the strength to get up
and search for the light and release the negativity from your mind and soul!

You start to cry as you find the strength to push despite feeling weak,
and your mind is releasing negativity and letting go of the past story.

A breakthrough is near as you start replenishing your mind with
positivity and optimism, and then suddenly, a smile graces your face.

This smile creates a ray of light that suddenly opens the
visual field and the path towards the light.

You shake off the debris as you slowly rise and
make your way to a recognizable place.

A place you needed to run from just for a moment, but
it's time to clean up and start living again.

You realize its easy to give up but more rewarding to
rise above the darkness and into the light.

Follow the sun and walk the path created for you.

The path will have some bumps, curves, mystery, and unexpected
popups, but keep your head high and look towards the sky,
the bright sun, and the moon to keep you afloat.

Happiness

What is happiness, and how does one obtain or feel the true meaning of happiness?

Is happiness due to continuing success, achievement, and delusions of a perfect life?

Or is happiness overcoming challenges, moving past obstacles,
and standing tall after the storm is gone?

Is happiness measured by the number of individuals that surround you?

Or is happiness measured by the ability to smile alone or
with one person to call a friend or family member?

Is happiness only when good fortune comes to you, or is it when lousy luck comes?

Question: What is life without issues, obstacles, experiences, etc.?

A boring and unhappy one if you ask me!

So, what is happiness?

I define happiness as being at peace with yourself and your surroundings
and finding beauty and joy despite the mess and chaos.

Spirituality and Me

As a spiritual person, I believe that everything in the universe is interconnected.
The energies that surround us carry messages from the divine (God), which
can be transmitted through various mediums. It's important to be receptive to
these messages and to tune in to the ways that God communicates with us.

Being a spiritual individual, I firmly believe that there exists a deep interconnection
between every entity that exists in the universe. The energies that surround us
have the potential to carry messages from the divine (God) and these messages can
be transmitted through various mediums. It is extremely crucial to be receptive
to these messages and to tune in to the ways that God communicates with us.

Alignment and Positive Vibes

I can't believe how lucky I am today! The sun is shining, and the birds are singing, making me feel so joyful and alive. I'm just bursting with excitement for all the wonderful things that are coming my way. I feel so loved and blessed, and I know that everything is going to work out just perfectly. Life is truly amazing, and I am so grateful for every moment of it. Today is going to be an incredible day, and I can't wait to see what the universe has in store for me!

Who am I ? .

The question "Who am I?" is closely tied to my parents, who brought me into this world. My beginnings were filled with joy and contentment, but over time, things became chaotic, noisy and confusing. I felt lonely, but the lotus flower serves as a symbol for me. Just like the lotus flower, I have risen from the murky waters of my past, and I am blooming into a vibrant, multi-faceted individual. I see myself as a healer, just like how a flower can be medicinal.

As I move forward, I am determined to focus on my goals. This means avoiding distractions like phone calls, TV and social media. To stay on track, I make a list of tasks and stick to a schedule. However, I also know the importance of socializing, so I make time for that too. Ultimately, I am excited to embrace the next chapter of my life. I want to find my groove again and, perhaps, even find love

A Seeker's Mission

*I'm on a mission to discover the truth and understand everything there is
to know about myself, the universe, and how everything is interconnected.
It's a big task, but I'm excited to explore and learn more daily!*

A seeker is a person who searches for something

or tries to find or obtain something:

Peace, understanding

*I am searching for truth and a deeper understanding of myself, the universe, and the
connections between things. As an investigator, explorer, and seeker, I am on a mission
to uncover the truth and gain knowledge about the things that surround me. Though
it is a daunting task, I am eager to explore and learn something new every day.*

*A big shoutout to my soul sister, Kerresha, for inspiring my recent
two pieces of writing, "Who am I" and "Seeker's Mission".* 😃

Contact information: Wholesome Touch

Website: www.wholesometouch.net

Email: Kproctor@wholesometouch.net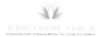

Tel: 📞 551-502-0273

REFERENCES

Bailey R. R. (2017). Goal Setting and Action Planning for Health Behavior Change. *American journal of lifestyle medicine*, *13*(6), 615–618. https://doi.org/10.1177/1559827617729634

Szabo, S., Tache, Y., & Somogyi, A. (2012). The legacy of Hans Selye and the origins of stress research: a retrospective 75 years after his landmark brief "letter" to the editor# of nature. *Stress (Amsterdam, Netherlands)*, *15*(5), 472–478. https://doi.org/10.3109/10253890.2012.710919

Bożek, A., Nowak, P. F., & Blukacz, M. (2020). The Relationship Between Spirituality, Health-Related Behavior, and Psychological Well-Being. *Frontiers in psychology*, *11*, 1997. https://doi.org/10.3389/fpsyg.2020.01997

Gualdi-Russo, E., & Zaccagni, L. (2021). Physical Activity for Health and Wellness. *International journal of environmental research and public health*, *18*(15), 7823. https://doi.org/10.3390/ijerph18157823

Steele, L. (2020). Holistic Well-Being: Mental, Physical, and Spiritual. In: Leal Filho, W., Wall, T., Azul, A.M., Brandli, L., Özuyar, P.G. (eds) Good Health and Well-Being. Encyclopedia of the UN Sustainable Development Goals. Springer, Cham. https://doi.org/10.1007/978-3-319-95681-7_1

Wu G. Dietary protein intake and human health. Food Funct. 2016;7(3):1251-1265. doi:10.1039/c5fo01530h

Delimaris I. Adverse Effects Associated with Protein Intake above the Recommended Dietary Allowance for Adults. ISRN Nutr. 2013;2013:126929. Published 2013 Jul 18. doi:10.5402/2013/126929

Lonnie M, Hooker E, Brunstrom JM, et al. Protein for Life: Review of Optimal Protein Intake, Sustainable Dietary Sources and the Effect on Appetite in Ageing Adults. Nutrients. 2018;10(3):360. Published 2018 Mar 16. doi:10.3390/nu10030360

Ramar K, Malhotra RK, Carden KA, et al. Sleep is essential to health: an American Academy of Sleep Medicine position statement. J Clin Sleep Med. 2021;17(10):2115–2119.

Braun L, Cohen M. *Herbs and Natural Supplements: An Evidence-Based Guide.* 4th ed. Volume 2. Elsevier; 2014.

Width M, Reinhard T. *The Essential Pocket Guide for Clinical Nutrition.* 3rd ed. Jones & Bartlett Learning; 2020.

Rakel DP. *Integrative Medicine.* 4th ed. Elsevier; 2018.

Hoffmann D. *Medical Herbalism: The Science and Practice of Herbal Medicine.* Simon and Schuster; 2003.

Weatherby D. *Signs and Symptoms Analysis from a Functional Perspective.* Weatherby & Associates, LLC; 2004

Printed in the USA
CPSIA information can be obtained
at www.ICGtesting.com
CBHW042012091024
15572CB00003B/48